This publication is intended to provide educational information for the reader on the covered subjects. It is not intended to take the place of personalized medical counseling, diagnosis, and treatment from a trained healthcare professional.

ISBN 978-1-998455-99-7 (Paperback)
ISBN 978-1-998740-00-0 (eBook)

Printed and bound in USA
Published by Loons Press

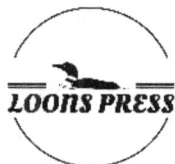

I0106308

LOONS PRESS

Table Of Contents

How To Prevent Pulmonary Embolism

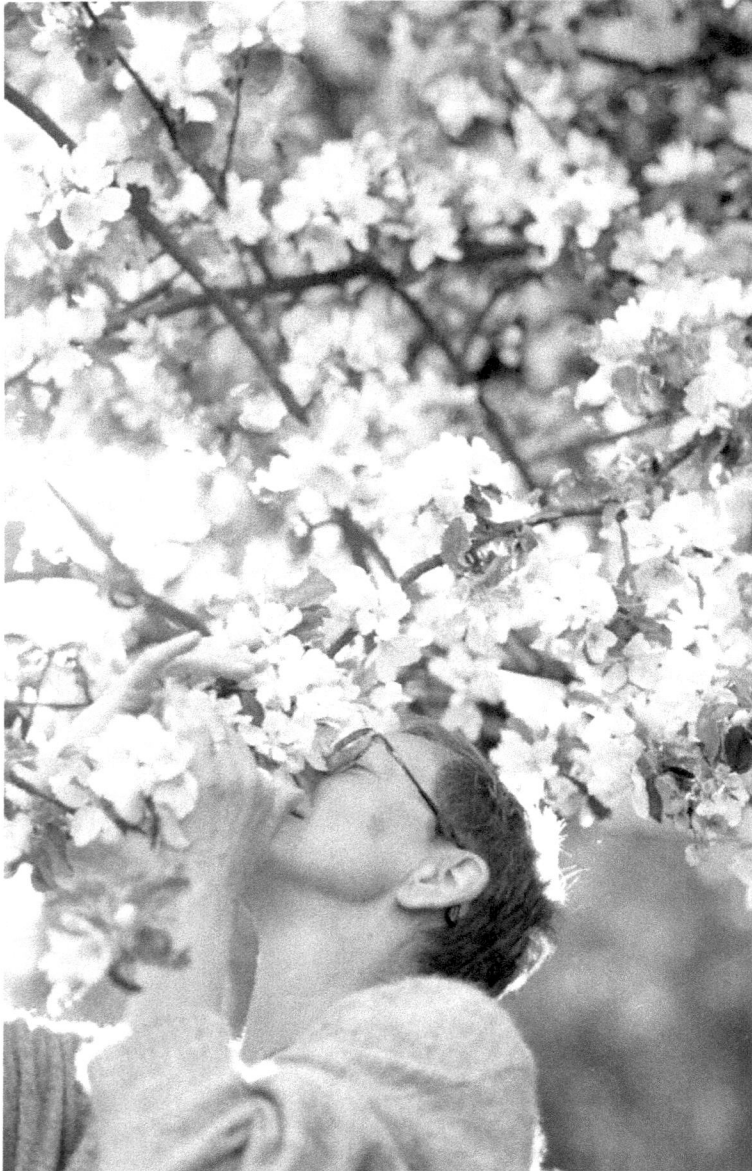

Chapter 1

Understanding Pulmonary Embolism

What is Pulmonary Embolism?

Pulmonary embolism (PE) is a serious medical condition that occurs when a blood clot blocks one or more arteries in the lungs. This blockage can significantly reduce blood flow to the lung tissue, leading to various complications.

The most common source of these blood clots is deep vein thrombosis (DVT), where clots form in the deep veins of the legs or other parts of the body and then travel to the lungs.

Understanding the nature of pulmonary embolism is crucial for recognizing its potential dangers and taking preventive measures.

The symptoms of pulmonary embolism can vary widely, ranging from mild to life-threatening. Common signs include sudden shortness of breath, chest pain that may worsen with deep breaths, rapid heart rate, and coughing up blood. Some individuals may experience anxiety or a feeling of impending doom. Because these symptoms can mimic those of other conditions, such as a heart attack or anxiety attack, it is essential to seek medical attention promptly if they occur. Early diagnosis and treatment can significantly improve outcomes.

Risk factors for developing pulmonary embolism include prolonged immobility, certain medical conditions, and lifestyle choices. Individuals who have undergone recent surgery, particularly orthopedic procedures, or those who are on long flights without movement are at increased risk.

Other contributing factors include obesity, smoking, hormonal therapies, and a personal or family history of blood clots. Being aware of these risk factors can empower individuals to take proactive steps in their health management.

Diagnosis of pulmonary embolism typically involves imaging tests, such as a computed tomography (CT) pulmonary angiogram or a ventilation-perfusion (V/Q) scan. Blood tests, including D-dimer tests, may also be performed to assess the likelihood of clot formation.

Once diagnosed, treatment options vary based on the severity of the PE and might include anticoagulants, thrombolytics, or, in severe cases, surgical interventions to remove the clot. Understanding the diagnostic process can help individuals navigate their healthcare journey more effectively.

Preventing pulmonary embolism is a multifaceted approach that includes lifestyle modifications and medical interventions. Regular physical activity, maintaining a healthy weight, staying hydrated, and avoiding prolonged periods of immobility are fundamental strategies. For those at high risk, healthcare providers may recommend prophylactic measures, such as blood thinners or compression stockings.

Educating oneself about pulmonary embolism and its prevention can significantly contribute to better lung health and overall well-being.

Risk Factors for Pulmonary Embolism

Pulmonary embolism (PE) is a serious condition that occurs when a blood clot blocks a pulmonary artery in the lungs, leading to potentially life-threatening consequences. Understanding the risk factors that contribute to the development of pulmonary embolism is crucial for prevention.

Several factors can increase an individual's likelihood of experiencing a PE, including age, underlying health conditions, and lifestyle choices. By recognizing these risk factors, individuals can take proactive steps to reduce their chances of developing this dangerous condition.

Age plays a significant role in the risk of pulmonary embolism. As individuals grow older, their blood vessels and circulatory system undergo changes that can predispose them to clot formation.

People over the age of 60 are particularly at higher risk, as the likelihood of developing conditions such as deep vein thrombosis (DVT) increases with age. Additionally, age-related immobility or decreased physical activity can further elevate the risk, making regular exercise and mobility essential for maintaining vascular health.

Certain medical conditions also heighten the risk of pulmonary embolism. These include heart diseases, cancer, and chronic respiratory conditions. For instance, patients with heart failure may experience poor circulation, leading to the formation of blood clots. Similarly, cancer patients are at an increased risk due to both the disease itself and the treatments, such as chemotherapy, which can affect blood clotting mechanisms.

Understanding these associations can empower individuals with these conditions to work closely with their healthcare providers to manage their health proactively.

Lifestyle choices significantly influence the risk of developing pulmonary embolism. Factors such as obesity, smoking, and prolonged periods of immobility can contribute to the likelihood of clot formation. Obesity increases pressure on the veins in the legs, while smoking can damage blood vessels and promote clotting.

Additionally, long periods of sitting, whether during travel or sedentary work, can impede blood flow and lead to DVT. Adopting a healthier lifestyle that includes regular physical activity, a balanced diet, and quitting smoking can drastically reduce the risk of PE.

Finally, certain medications and genetic predispositions can also increase the risk of pulmonary embolism. Hormonal therapies, including birth control pills and hormone replacement therapy, may elevate the risk of clot formation, particularly in women who smoke or have other risk factors. Additionally, genetic conditions such as Factor V Leiden mutation can predispose individuals to develop blood clots more easily.

Awareness of these factors allows individuals to consult healthcare professionals about alternative options or monitoring strategies to mitigate their risk, ultimately leading to better lung health and overall well-being.

Symptoms of Pulmonary Embolism

Pulmonary embolism (PE) is a serious condition that occurs when a blood clot blocks a blood vessel in the lungs, leading to potentially life-threatening consequences. Recognizing the symptoms of pulmonary embolism is crucial for timely intervention and effective treatment. The symptoms can vary significantly from person to person, making awareness and knowledge essential for those at risk.

One of the most common symptoms of pulmonary embolism is sudden shortness of breath. This may occur unexpectedly and can range from mild to severe. Individuals might feel as though they cannot catch their breath or may experience a sense of anxiety as their breathing changes. In some cases, this shortness of breath may worsen with physical activity or when lying down, prompting individuals to seek immediate medical attention.

Chest pain is another prominent symptom associated with pulmonary embolism. The pain can be sharp or dull and may resemble that of a heart attack, often described as a feeling of pressure or tightness. This discomfort may also radiate to the shoulder, arm, neck, or jaw.

Patients may notice that the pain intensifies with deep breaths, coughs, or movements, which can lead to further distress and the need for urgent medical evaluation.

Coughing, particularly if it is accompanied by blood-streaked sputum, is also a significant warning sign of pulmonary embolism. While a cough can be attributed to various conditions, the presence of blood or a sudden change in the nature of the cough should alert individuals to the possibility of a serious underlying issue.

Other symptoms may include rapid heart rate and lightheadedness, which can accompany the sudden onset of pulmonary embolism and may indicate a decrease in oxygen levels in the bloodstream.

In addition to the more commonly recognized symptoms, less obvious signs such as swelling in one leg, particularly in the calf, may also occur due to deep vein thrombosis, a condition that often precedes pulmonary embolism. This swelling can be accompanied by warmth, redness, or tenderness in the affected area. Recognizing these symptoms is vital, as leg swelling can often be overlooked or misdiagnosed, delaying the diagnosis and treatment of pulmonary embolism.

Understanding and identifying the symptoms of pulmonary embolism can significantly impact outcomes for those at risk. Prompt recognition and seeking medical assistance can be lifesaving.

It is essential for individuals to remain vigilant about their health, especially if they have risk factors for venous thromboembolism, such as prolonged immobility, recent surgery, or a history of clotting disorders. By educating themselves about the signs and symptoms, individuals can take proactive steps towards better lung health and prevention of pulmonary embolism.

Diagnosis of Pulmonary Embolism

Diagnosis of pulmonary embolism (PE) is a critical step in managing this potentially life-threatening condition. The symptoms of PE can often mimic those of other respiratory or cardiovascular issues, making accurate diagnosis essential. Common symptoms include sudden shortness of breath, chest pain that may worsen with deep breathing, coughing up blood, and rapid heart rate.

However, these symptoms can also be associated with anxiety, pneumonia, or heart conditions, which complicates the diagnostic process. Therefore, a thorough medical history and physical examination by a healthcare professional are crucial for distinguishing PE from these other conditions.

To confirm a diagnosis of pulmonary embolism, healthcare providers utilize a variety of imaging techniques. The most commonly used test is the computed tomography pulmonary angiography (CTPA), which provides detailed images of the blood vessels in the lungs. CTPA is highly effective in visualizing clots within these vessels and is considered the gold standard for PE diagnosis.

Additionally, a ventilation-perfusion (V/Q) scan may be employed when a CTPA is contraindicated or when patients have renal issues that prevent the use of contrast material. This scan evaluates the airflow and blood flow in the lungs, helping to identify areas that are not receiving adequate blood flow due to a blockage.

In some cases, blood tests are also utilized to aid in the diagnosis of pulmonary embolism. The D-dimer test measures the presence of a substance in the blood that is released when a blood clot breaks down. Elevated levels of D-dimer can indicate the presence of an abnormal clot, but this test is not specific to PE and can be elevated in other conditions as well.

Therefore, while a negative D-dimer test can help rule out PE, a positive result often necessitates further imaging studies for confirmation. The combination of clinical assessment, imaging, and laboratory tests creates a comprehensive approach to diagnosing pulmonary embolism.

In certain situations, additional diagnostic tools may be employed, particularly in patients with atypical presentations or those who have a high risk for complications. For example, an echocardiogram can be useful in assessing the heart's function and detecting right ventricular strain, which may occur in cases of significant pulmonary embolism.

Invasive procedures, such as pulmonary angiography, may also be considered in complex cases, particularly when interventional treatment is being planned. This tailored approach to diagnosis ensures that patients receive the most appropriate and timely care based on their individual risk factors and clinical presentation.

Understanding the diagnostic process for pulmonary embolism is vital for individuals concerned about their lung health. Recognizing the symptoms and seeking prompt medical attention can significantly improve outcomes. Furthermore, awareness of the diagnostic methods used can empower patients to engage in informed discussions with their healthcare providers.

By prioritizing early diagnosis and intervention, individuals can take proactive steps toward preventing the serious complications associated with pulmonary embolism, ultimately enhancing their overall lung health and well-being.

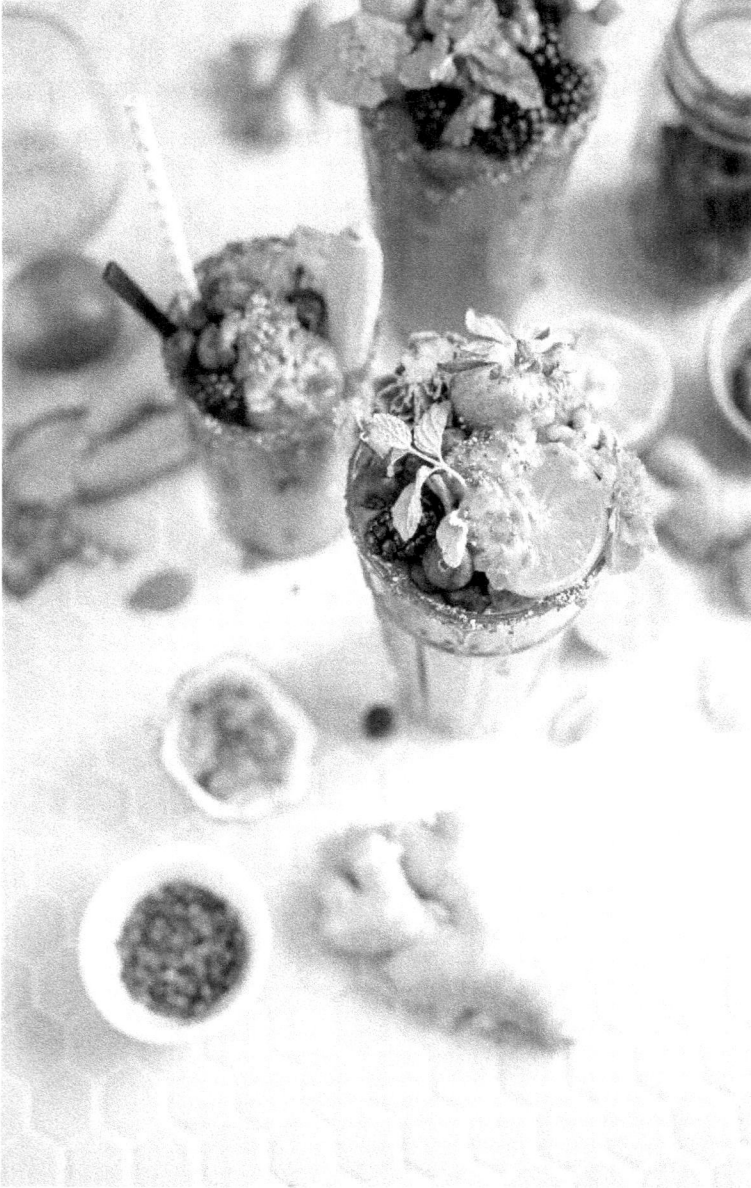

Chapter 2

The Importance of Prevention

Why Prevention Matters

Prevention plays a crucial role in reducing the incidence and impact of pulmonary embolism (PE), a serious condition that can lead to severe health complications and even death. Understanding the importance of preventive measures empowers individuals to take charge of their health and make informed choices. By recognizing the risk factors associated with PE and adopting strategies to mitigate them, individuals can significantly lower their chances of experiencing this life-threatening event.

One of the primary reasons prevention matters is that pulmonary embolism often occurs without warning and may present with vague symptoms that can be easily overlooked. Many individuals do not realize they are at risk until it is too late.

By educating oneself about the risk factors, such as prolonged immobility, obesity, and certain medical conditions, individuals can remain vigilant and proactive. This awareness enables early intervention and lifestyle adjustments that can prevent the formation of blood clots, which are the primary culprits behind PE.

Another critical aspect of prevention is the impact on overall health and well-being. Engaging in regular physical activity, maintaining a healthy weight, and adhering to prescribed medical treatments can enhance cardiovascular health and improve circulation.

These lifestyle choices not only reduce the risk of pulmonary embolism but also contribute to a lower likelihood of other related health issues, such as deep vein thrombosis. By prioritizing preventive measures, individuals can foster a holistic approach to their health, leading to a better quality of life.

Additionally, the financial implications of pulmonary embolism can be significant. Treating a PE often requires extensive medical intervention, including hospitalization, diagnostic imaging, and long-term medication. These costs can strain personal finances and healthcare systems alike. By focusing on prevention, individuals can avoid the potentially overwhelming expenses associated with treating a PE. Investing time and resources into preventive strategies ultimately pays off in both health and financial terms.

Finally, fostering a culture of prevention within communities can enhance public health outcomes. When individuals prioritize prevention and share their knowledge and experiences, it creates a ripple effect that encourages others to do the same. Community education programs, support groups, and healthcare initiatives can amplify awareness of pulmonary embolism and the importance of prevention.

By working together, communities can significantly reduce the prevalence of this condition, leading to healthier populations and enhanced quality of life for all.

The Impact of Lifestyle on Lung Health

Lifestyle choices play a crucial role in determining overall lung health and can significantly influence the risk of developing conditions like pulmonary embolism. The lungs are vital organs that require optimal care to function effectively. Factors such as diet, physical activity, smoking, and stress management directly affect lung capacity and respiratory function.

Understanding these elements allows individuals to make informed decisions that enhance lung health and reduce the likelihood of serious complications.

A balanced diet rich in fruits, vegetables, whole grains, and lean proteins can greatly benefit lung function. Antioxidants found in various foods help combat oxidative stress, which can damage lung tissue. Omega-3 fatty acids, prevalent in fish and nuts, have anti-inflammatory properties that may also protect lung health.

Staying hydrated is equally important, as adequate fluid intake helps maintain mucosal linings in the respiratory tract, facilitating easier breathing and reducing the risk of infections that could lead to complications like pulmonary embolism.

Regular physical activity is another key component of a lung-friendly lifestyle. Engaging in aerobic exercises such as walking, running, or cycling can improve cardiovascular health and enhance lung capacity. Exercise promotes better circulation, which is vital for preventing blood clots that can lead to pulmonary embolism.

Additionally, activities such as yoga and deep-breathing exercises can improve lung function by increasing respiratory efficiency and reducing stress, which in turn can lower the risk of clot formation.

Conversely, smoking is one of the most detrimental lifestyle choices for lung health. It not only damages lung tissue but also increases the likelihood of chronic respiratory diseases that can heighten the risk of pulmonary embolism.

Quitting smoking can lead to significant improvements in lung function over time, reducing inflammation and allowing the lungs to heal. Furthermore, avoiding secondhand smoke is crucial, as it exposes non-smokers to similar risks associated with direct tobacco use.

Stress management cannot be overlooked when discussing lung health. Chronic stress can lead to shallow breathing and increased tension in the body, which may negatively impact lung function. Techniques such as mindfulness, meditation, and relaxation exercises can help manage stress effectively.

By promoting a calm state of mind, individuals can improve their breathing patterns and overall lung health, thereby lowering the risk of developing conditions that could lead to pulmonary embolism. Making conscious lifestyle choices is essential for maintaining optimal lung health and preventing serious complications.

Understanding the Burden of Pulmonary Embolism

Pulmonary embolism (PE) is a serious health condition that occurs when a blood clot travels to the lungs, blocking a pulmonary artery. This blockage can lead to significant complications, including damage to the lung and reduced oxygen levels in the bloodstream.

Understanding the burden of pulmonary embolism is crucial for individuals concerned about their lung health, as it highlights the importance of prevention and awareness. The impact of PE can be profound, not only physically but also emotionally and financially, making it essential to recognize the signs and risks associated with this condition.

One of the main contributors to pulmonary embolism is deep vein thrombosis (DVT), where blood clots form in the deep veins of the legs. If these clots dislodge, they can travel to the lungs and cause a PE.

The symptoms of a pulmonary embolism can vary significantly, sometimes presenting as sudden shortness of breath, chest pain, or even coughing up blood. These symptoms can be easily mistaken for other conditions, which can delay diagnosis and treatment. Early recognition is vital to mitigate the effects of PE, as timely medical intervention can be life-saving.

The burden of pulmonary embolism extends beyond immediate health concerns. Individuals who experience a PE may face long-term complications, including chronic pulmonary hypertension or reduced exercise capacity. These complications can lead to a decreased quality of life, affecting daily activities and contributing to anxiety and depression.

Furthermore, the fear of recurrent episodes can create a psychological burden, leading individuals to alter their lifestyles and limit their activities out of concern for their health.

Financially, the impact of pulmonary embolism can be significant. The costs associated with emergency care, hospitalization, and potential long-term management of complications can be overwhelming. Additionally, individuals may face lost income due to inability to work during recovery.

This financial strain can exacerbate the emotional burden, leading to a cycle of stress and health deterioration. Understanding these potential costs can motivate individuals to prioritize preventive measures and seek timely medical advice.

Awareness and education about pulmonary embolism are critical components in alleviating its burden. Individuals can take proactive steps to reduce their risk, including regular physical activity, maintaining a healthy weight, and staying hydrated, especially during long periods of immobility.

Knowing the risk factors, such as recent surgery, prolonged bed rest, or certain medical conditions, can empower individuals to advocate for their health.

By fostering a greater understanding of pulmonary embolism and its impacts, individuals can better navigate their path to improved lung health and overall well-being.

How To Prevent Pulmonary Embolism

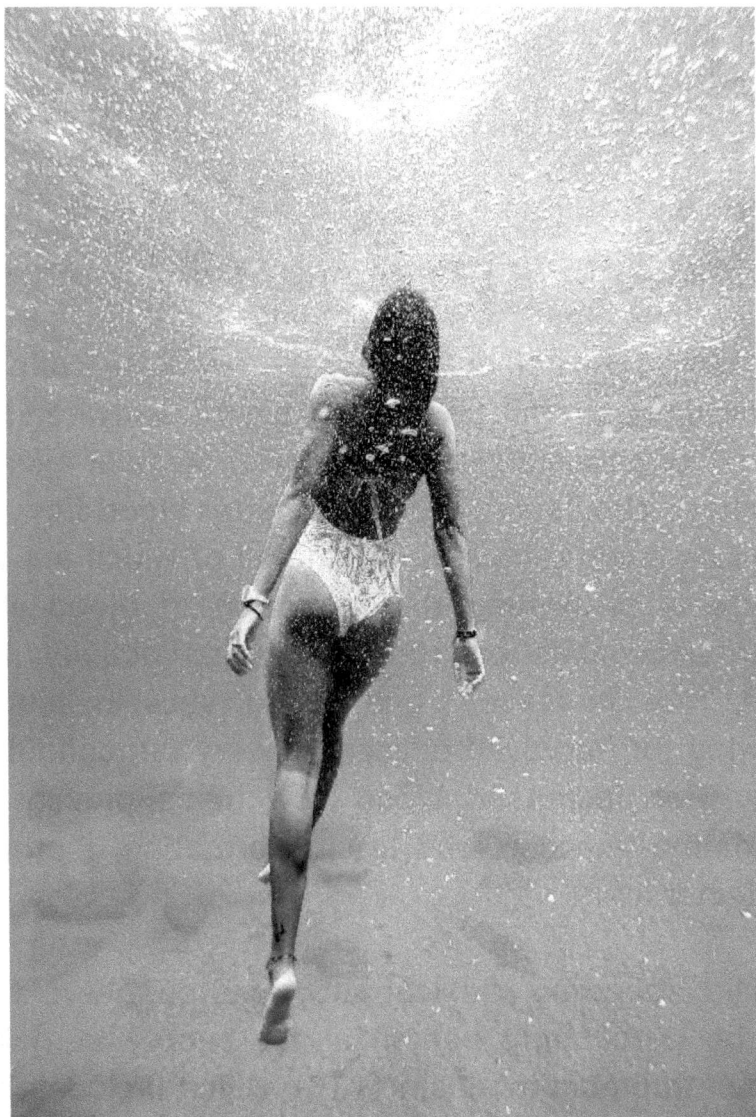

Your Path to Better Lung Health

Chapter 3

Lifestyle Modifications

The Role of Physical Activity

Physical activity plays a crucial role in maintaining overall health and significantly reducing the risk of pulmonary embolism (PE). Regular exercise enhances circulation, promotes better blood flow, and helps maintain a healthy weight, all of which are vital factors in preventing the formation of blood clots. When individuals engage in physical activity, their heart rate increases, and blood vessels expand, allowing for improved oxygen delivery throughout the body. This increased blood flow helps prevent the stagnation that can lead to clot formation, a primary risk factor for PE.

Incorporating physical activity into daily routines can be particularly beneficial for people at risk of venous thromboembolism (VTE), which includes both deep vein thrombosis (DVT) and pulmonary embolism.

Activities such as walking, swimming, cycling, and even stretching can be effective in keeping the blood flowing. For those with sedentary lifestyles or occupations that require long periods of sitting, taking regular breaks to stand up, stretch, or walk can make a significant difference in reducing the likelihood of clot development. The key is to find activities that are enjoyable and sustainable, making it easier to establish a consistent routine.

Furthermore, strength training exercises can also play an important role in enhancing muscle tone and improving overall physical fitness. Stronger muscles support better circulation and assist in the movement of blood back to the heart.

Engaging in resistance training two to three times a week can complement aerobic activities and contribute to better cardiovascular health. It is essential, however, to start slowly and gradually increase the intensity and duration of workouts, especially for individuals who may not have been physically active for some time.

In addition to the physical benefits, regular exercise has positive effects on mental health, which can indirectly influence the risk of pulmonary embolism. Stress, anxiety, and depression can lead to unhealthy lifestyle choices, such as poor diet or inactivity, which can increase the risk of developing blood clots.

Physical activity releases endorphins, which improve mood and can help individuals manage stress more effectively. By fostering a positive mental state, individuals are more likely to engage in healthy behaviors that support their overall well-being and reduce the risk of PE.

Lastly, it is important to consult with a healthcare provider before starting any new exercise regimen, especially for individuals with existing health conditions or those who have previously experienced blood clots. Tailoring a physical activity plan to individual needs and limitations ensures safety and maximizes the health benefits. By understanding the vital role of physical activity in preventing pulmonary embolism, individuals can take proactive steps toward improving their lung health and overall quality of life.

Nutrition for Optimal Lung Health

Nutrition plays a crucial role in maintaining optimal lung health and can significantly influence the risk of developing conditions like pulmonary embolism. A balanced diet rich in essential nutrients supports the respiratory system and enhances overall well-being. Key nutrients such as antioxidants, vitamins, and minerals can help reduce inflammation, strengthen lung function, and improve blood circulation, which is vital in preventing blood clots that lead to pulmonary embolism.

Understanding how specific foods and dietary patterns contribute to lung health can empower individuals to make healthier choices.

Antioxidants are particularly beneficial for lung health as they combat oxidative stress caused by free radicals. Foods high in antioxidants, such as berries, leafy greens, nuts, and seeds, can help protect lung tissue from damage. Vitamin C, found in citrus fruits, bell peppers, and broccoli, is known for its immune-boosting properties and its ability to improve lung function.

Similarly, vitamin E, present in almonds, sunflower seeds, and avocados, contributes to maintaining healthy lung tissue. Incorporating a variety of these antioxidant-rich foods into daily meals can provide the necessary support for optimal lung health.

Omega-3 fatty acids are another vital component of a lung-healthy diet. These healthy fats, found in fatty fish like salmon, flaxseeds, and walnuts, possess anti-inflammatory properties that can help reduce lung inflammation. Chronic inflammation is a risk factor for various respiratory diseases and may contribute to the development of blood clots. By including omega-3-rich foods in the diet, individuals can promote better lung function and reduce their risk of complications related to pulmonary embolism.

Hydration is an often-overlooked aspect of nutrition that is essential for lung health. Proper hydration helps maintain the mucosal lining of the airways, which is crucial for trapping allergens and pathogens. It also helps thin mucus secretions, making it easier to expel.

Drinking an adequate amount of water daily, along with herbal teas and other hydrating fluids, supports the overall function of the respiratory system.

Staying hydrated is particularly important for individuals who may be at risk of blood clot formation, as adequate fluid intake promotes healthy blood circulation.

In addition to specific nutrients, adopting a balanced eating pattern is important for maintaining lung health. Diets rich in whole grains, lean proteins, fruits, and vegetables can provide the necessary nutrients without excess calories or unhealthy fats. Limiting processed foods, refined sugars, and trans fats can also help reduce inflammation and improve overall health.

By making informed dietary choices and focusing on nutrient-dense foods, individuals can create a supportive environment for their lungs, ultimately reducing the risk of pulmonary embolism and enhancing their quality of life.

Importance of Hydration

Hydration plays a critical role in maintaining overall health, particularly for individuals concerned about pulmonary embolism. Proper hydration ensures that the blood remains at an optimal viscosity, which is essential for preventing clot formation. When the body is well-hydrated, blood flows more freely through the veins and arteries, reducing the risk of stagnation that can contribute to the development of clots. For individuals with existing health concerns or those at higher risk of pulmonary embolism, understanding the importance of adequate fluid intake is paramount.

The human body requires a certain amount of fluid daily to function correctly, with recommendations typically ranging from 8 to 10 cups for the average adult. However, this requirement can vary depending on factors such as age, activity level, and climate. When the body is not sufficiently hydrated, the blood can become thicker, making it more prone to clotting.

This thickening can be particularly dangerous for those with conditions that already predispose them to clot formation, as it increases the likelihood of a pulmonary embolism.

In addition to supporting healthy blood viscosity, hydration also aids in the proper functioning of the circulatory system. Water helps to transport oxygen and nutrients throughout the body while facilitating waste removal. When the body is dehydrated, these processes can become impaired, leading to a range of health issues.

For those concerned about pulmonary embolism, maintaining hydration is vital not only for blood health but also for overall respiratory function, as the body's tissues require adequate hydration to operate effectively.

Moreover, hydration plays a significant role in physical activity and recovery. For individuals at risk of pulmonary embolism, engaging in regular, moderate exercise is often recommended to promote circulation. However, physical activity increases the body's demand for fluids. Dehydration during exercise can lead to fatigue, dizziness, and even impaired cognitive function, all of which may hinder an individual's ability to maintain an active lifestyle that supports vascular health. Ensuring proper hydration before, during, and after physical activity can help mitigate these risks.

Ultimately, understanding the importance of hydration is a key component in preventing pulmonary embolism. Individuals should prioritize fluid intake as part of their daily routine, particularly if they have risk factors associated with clot formation.

Simple strategies such as carrying a water bottle, setting reminders to drink, and incorporating hydrating foods into meals can help maintain adequate hydration levels. By fostering a proactive approach to hydration, individuals can significantly enhance their lung health and reduce the risk of serious complications associated with pulmonary embolism.

Weight Management Strategies

Weight management plays a crucial role in reducing the risk of pulmonary embolism, as excess weight can increase the likelihood of blood clots forming in the body. Maintaining a healthy weight can improve overall cardiovascular health, enhance mobility, and reduce pressure on the veins, particularly in the lower extremities.

Individuals who are overweight or obese are at a greater risk of developing deep vein thrombosis, which can lead to pulmonary embolism if a clot dislodges and travels to the lungs. Therefore, adopting effective weight management strategies is essential for anyone concerned about pulmonary embolism.

A balanced diet is the cornerstone of effective weight management. Incorporating a variety of fruits, vegetables, whole grains, lean proteins, and healthy fats can help individuals achieve and maintain a healthy weight. It is important to focus on portion control and mindful eating practices, as overeating can contribute to weight gain. Additionally, reducing the intake of processed foods, sugary beverages, and high-calorie snacks can significantly support weight loss efforts. Keeping a food diary may also help individuals track their eating habits and make more informed choices.

Regular physical activity is another vital component of weight management. Engaging in aerobic exercises, such as walking, cycling, or swimming, can help burn calories and improve cardiovascular health.

Strength training is also beneficial, as it builds muscle mass, which can increase metabolism and aid in weight loss. Aim for at least 150 minutes of moderate-intensity exercise each week, combined with muscle-strengthening activities on two or more days. This not only helps in weight management but also enhances circulation, reducing the risk of clot formation.

Behavioral strategies can also enhance weight management efforts. Setting realistic goals, such as losing 1-2 pounds per week, can lead to sustainable weight loss. Finding a support system, whether through friends, family, or support groups, can provide motivation and accountability.

Additionally, addressing emotional eating by developing healthier coping mechanisms can prevent weight gain. Mindfulness practices, such as meditation or yoga, can help in recognizing emotional triggers and improving overall mental well-being, which is closely linked to physical health.

Finally, it is essential to consult healthcare professionals when implementing weight management strategies. A registered dietitian can provide personalized guidance on nutrition, while a fitness trainer can design an effective exercise regimen tailored to individual needs and capabilities. Regular check-ins with healthcare providers can help monitor progress and make necessary adjustments to weight management plans.

By prioritizing weight management through these strategies, individuals can significantly reduce their risk of pulmonary embolism and improve their overall lung health.

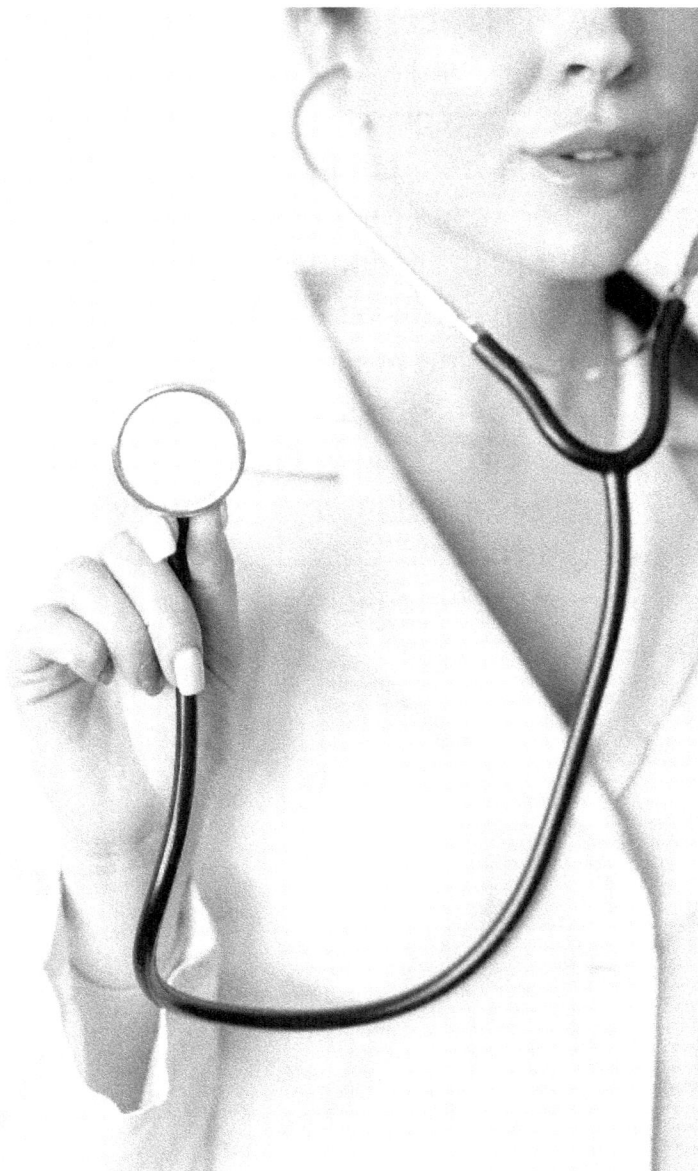

Chapter 4
Medical Interventions

Understanding Anticoagulants

Anticoagulants, commonly referred to as blood thinners, play a critical role in preventing the formation of blood clots that can lead to serious complications such as pulmonary embolism. These medications work by disrupting the blood clotting process, which is essential for maintaining proper circulation and preventing excessive bleeding. Understanding how anticoagulants function can empower individuals to make informed decisions about their health and enhance their preventive strategies against conditions that may result in pulmonary embolism.

There are several types of anticoagulants, each with distinct mechanisms of action. The most commonly prescribed anticoagulants include warfarin, direct oral anticoagulants (DOACs) like rivaroxaban and apixaban, and low molecular weight heparins such as enoxaparin.

Warfarin requires regular blood monitoring to ensure therapeutic levels are maintained, while DOACs offer the advantage of fixed dosing without the need for routine blood tests. Low molecular weight heparins are often administered via injection and are frequently used in hospital settings for immediate anticoagulation.

The choice of anticoagulant depends on various factors, including the patient's medical history, the risk of clot formation, and potential interactions with other medications. Physicians consider these elements to tailor a treatment plan that minimizes the risk of pulmonary embolism while also balancing the potential for bleeding complications. It is crucial for patients to communicate openly with their healthcare providers about any existing conditions, medications, or lifestyle factors that may influence their anticoagulant therapy.

While anticoagulants are effective in reducing the risk of pulmonary embolism, they are not without risks. Patients must be aware of the signs of excessive bleeding, such as unusual bruising, prolonged bleeding from cuts, or blood in urine or stool.

Additionally, lifestyle modifications, such as maintaining a healthy diet, managing weight, and avoiding activities that increase the risk of injury, can further enhance the safety and efficacy of anticoagulant therapy. Regular follow-ups with healthcare providers are essential to monitor the treatment's effectiveness and make necessary adjustments.

In summary, understanding anticoagulants is vital for individuals concerned about pulmonary embolism. Knowledge of the different types of anticoagulants, their mechanisms, and their associated risks can help patients engage actively in their treatment plans.

By working closely with healthcare professionals and adhering to prescribed therapies, patients can significantly reduce their risk of developing blood clots and improve their overall lung health.

When to Consider Compression Stockings

Compression stockings are a valuable tool for individuals seeking to prevent pulmonary embolism, particularly for those at risk due to prolonged periods of immobility or underlying medical conditions. Understanding when to consider wearing these stockings can significantly enhance your strategy for maintaining optimal vascular health.

Compression stockings work by applying graduated pressure to the legs, which helps improve blood flow and prevent the pooling of blood in the veins. This is especially crucial for individuals with a history of deep vein thrombosis (DVT) or those who have undergone recent surgical procedures.

One primary scenario where compression stockings are advisable is during long periods of travel. Individuals embarking on long flights or car rides may experience decreased blood circulation due to extended immobility.

The risk of DVT, which can lead to pulmonary embolism if a clot dislodges, increases significantly in these situations. Wearing compression stockings during travel can mitigate this risk by promoting better venous return and reducing swelling, making them an essential accessory for frequent travelers or those undertaking long journeys.

Additionally, individuals recovering from surgery, particularly orthopedic or abdominal surgeries, should consider using compression stockings. Post-surgical patients are often immobilized for extended periods, which heightens their risk for clot formation.

Compression stockings can play a crucial role in their recovery process by maintaining blood circulation in the legs, minimizing swelling, and promoting healing. Surgeons frequently recommend these stockings as part of the post-operative care plan to optimize recovery and prevent complications such as DVT and subsequent pulmonary embolism.

For those with medical conditions such as obesity, chronic venous insufficiency, or varicose veins, the use of compression stockings can be particularly beneficial. These conditions can impair blood flow and increase the likelihood of blood clots forming in the legs. Wearing compression stockings can help manage symptoms associated with these conditions while also providing preventive benefits against clot formation.

It is essential for individuals with such health concerns to consult with their healthcare provider to determine the appropriate type and level of compression needed to maximize benefits.

Lastly, individuals who lead sedentary lifestyles or have occupations that require prolonged sitting or standing should also consider incorporating compression stockings into their daily routine. Jobs that involve long hours at a desk or standing without frequent movement can contribute to poor circulation and increase the risk of DVT.

By wearing compression stockings, these individuals can support healthy blood flow, reduce discomfort, and ultimately lower the risk of developing complications that could lead to pulmonary embolism.

Regular movement, combined with the use of compression stockings, can provide an effective strategy for maintaining vascular health and preventing serious conditions.

The Role of Surgery in Prevention

Surgery plays a significant role in the prevention of pulmonary embolism (PE) for certain individuals who are at a heightened risk due to various medical conditions. Understanding the surgical options available can be vital for those concerned about PE, especially after experiencing risk factors such as deep vein thrombosis (DVT) or undergoing major surgery.

In some cases, surgical interventions can directly reduce the likelihood of blood clots forming or traveling to the lungs, ultimately decreasing the chances of a pulmonary embolism.

One of the primary surgical options for preventing PE is the placement of an inferior vena cava (IVC) filter. This device is inserted into the inferior vena cava, the large vein responsible for carrying blood from the lower body back to the heart. The IVC filter captures blood clots that may dislodge from the legs or pelvis before they can reach the lungs.

This procedure is particularly beneficial for patients who cannot take anticoagulant medications due to bleeding disorders or other contraindications. Understanding the criteria for IVC filter placement is essential for those at risk for DVT and subsequent PE.

In addition to IVC filters, surgical procedures may also involve the removal of existing clots. Thrombectomy, a procedure that involves the surgical removal of blood clots from the veins, can be performed in cases where a patient presents with significant DVT. By addressing the clot directly, this intervention can help restore normal blood flow and significantly reduce the risk of PE.

It is crucial for patients to discuss the potential benefits and risks of such procedures with their healthcare provider to determine the best course of action for their individual circumstances.

Preventive surgery is not limited to interventions aimed directly at blood clots. For individuals with specific medical conditions, such as certain cancers or hereditary clotting disorders, prophylactic surgeries may be recommended to reduce thrombotic events. For example, surgical removal of tumors that compress veins can improve venous return and decrease the risk of clot formation. Patients should engage in conversations with their healthcare team to explore all preventive measures, including lifestyle changes and surgical options, that may be appropriate for them.

Ultimately, the role of surgery in preventing pulmonary embolism is an important consideration for individuals at risk. While surgical interventions can provide significant benefits, they are typically part of a broader approach that includes medication management, lifestyle modifications, and regular monitoring.

By understanding the surgical options available and engaging with healthcare providers, individuals can take proactive steps to reduce their risk of PE and improve their overall lung health.

Regular Medical Check-Ups

Regular medical check-ups play a crucial role in maintaining overall health and preventing serious conditions such as pulmonary embolism. These check-ups provide an opportunity for healthcare providers to assess risk factors, monitor existing health issues, and offer guidance on lifestyle changes that can enhance lung health.

For individuals concerned about pulmonary embolism, proactive medical visits can significantly reduce the risk by ensuring that potential warning signs are identified and addressed early.

During regular check-ups, healthcare professionals typically review a patient's medical history, including any previous instances of blood clots, surgeries, or prolonged periods of immobility.

Understanding these risk factors is essential because they can contribute to the likelihood of developing deep vein thrombosis (DVT), which is a primary precursor to pulmonary embolism. By discussing personal and family medical histories, patients can work with their doctors to create a tailored prevention strategy that may include medication, lifestyle adjustments, or further diagnostic testing.

Physical examinations during these visits also allow healthcare providers to evaluate the patient's cardiovascular health. Monitoring blood pressure, heart rate, and overall circulation can provide critical insights into an individual's risk for clot formation.

In addition, doctors may recommend blood tests to assess clotting factors or check for conditions like atrial fibrillation, which can increase the likelihood of embolism. Regular monitoring can lead to timely interventions that help mitigate risks before they escalate into more serious health issues.

Furthermore, regular check-ups offer an excellent platform for discussing lifestyle factors that influence lung health. Healthcare providers can educate patients on the importance of maintaining a healthy weight, engaging in regular physical activity, and avoiding smoking. These lifestyle choices not only promote overall well-being but also significantly lower the risk of conditions that can lead to pulmonary embolism. Creating a dialogue about these factors during medical visits empowers patients to take an active role in their health management.

In summary, prioritizing regular medical check-ups is an essential step in preventing pulmonary embolism. These appointments facilitate open communication between patients and healthcare providers, enabling early detection and intervention for risk factors associated with blood clots.

By actively participating in their health care and adhering to medical advice, individuals can improve their lung health and reduce their chances of experiencing a potentially life-threatening pulmonary embolism.

How To Prevent Pulmonary Embolism

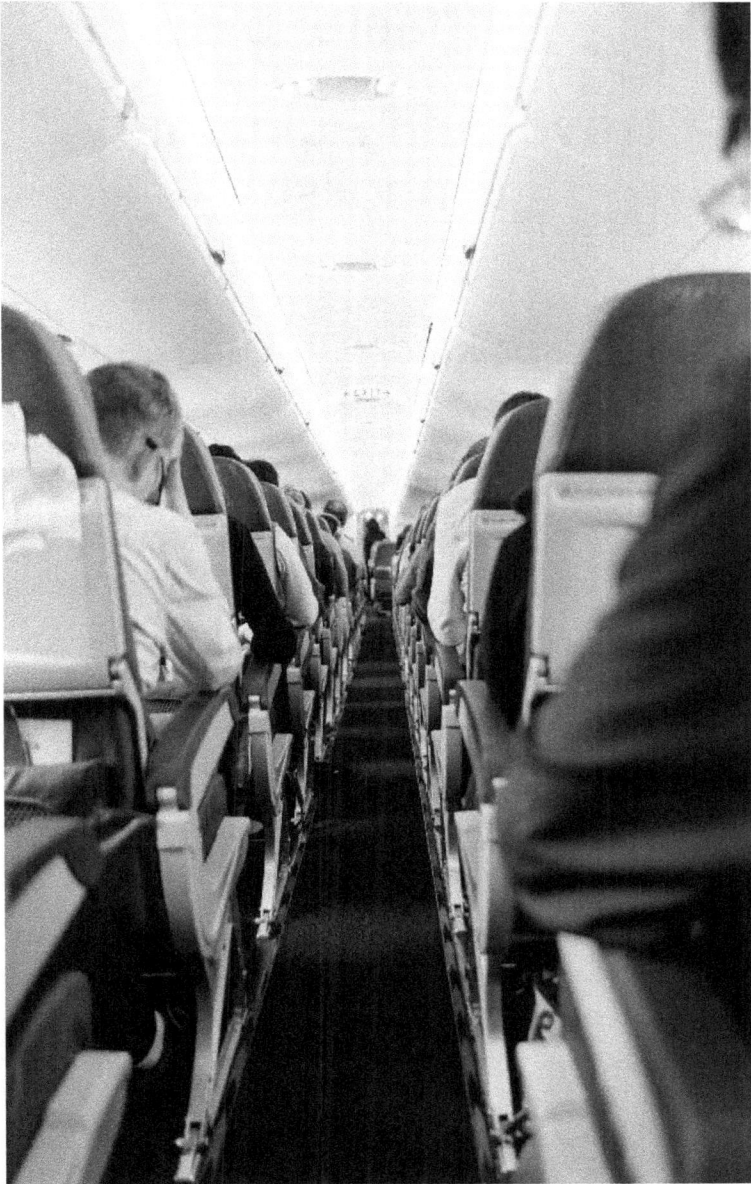

Chapter 5

Travel and Pulmonary Embolism

Risks Associated with Long-Distance Travel

Long-distance travel, whether by air, train, or car, poses specific risks that can significantly impact lung health and increase the likelihood of developing pulmonary embolism.

One of the primary concerns during extended periods of immobility is venous thromboembolism, a condition where blood clots form in the deep veins of the legs and can dislodge, traveling to the lungs.

This risk is heightened during long journeys, especially when individuals remain seated for prolonged periods without adequate movement.

Dehydration is another factor to consider during long-distance travel. Air travel, in particular, can lead to lower humidity levels in the cabin, causing dehydration that may affect blood viscosity.

When the blood becomes thicker, it is more prone to clotting. Travelers should be proactive in maintaining hydration by drinking plenty of fluids throughout their journey, avoiding excessive alcohol and caffeine consumption that can exacerbate dehydration.

Additionally, underlying health conditions can further elevate the risks associated with long-distance travel. Individuals with a history of clotting disorders, previous episodes of deep vein thrombosis, or those who are pregnant should take extra precautions.

Consulting a healthcare professional prior to traveling can provide personalized advice and preventive strategies tailored to individual health needs, ensuring that travelers are aware of their specific risks and how to mitigate them.

Wearing compression stockings is an effective strategy for reducing the risk of blood clots during long trips. These specially designed stockings promote blood circulation in the legs, minimizing the chances of clot formation.

Travelers should consider wearing compression stockings during flights or while driving for extended periods, as they can provide a significant barrier against the complications associated with immobility and poor circulation.

Finally, maintaining an active routine during travel can help combat the risks of pulmonary embolism. Taking regular breaks to walk around, stretching legs, and performing simple exercises can enhance blood flow and reduce the likelihood of clot formation. Integrating movement into travel plans is essential, as it not only supports lung health but also contributes to overall well-being during long journeys.

By being aware of these risks and implementing preventive measures, travelers can significantly lower the chances of experiencing complications such as pulmonary embolism.

Tips for Staying Active While Traveling

Traveling can pose unique challenges for individuals concerned about pulmonary embolism, particularly due to prolonged periods of inactivity. Staying active while on the move is essential for maintaining circulation and reducing the risk of blood clots.

To help you stay engaged in physical activity during your travels, consider incorporating simple strategies into your itinerary that promote movement without sacrificing enjoyment.

One effective way to remain active is to schedule regular breaks during long journeys. If you're traveling by plane, train, or car, make it a point to stand up, stretch, and walk around every hour or so. This practice encourages blood flow and reduces the risk of stagnant circulation.

When flying, take advantage of the opportunity to walk up and down the aisle, and perform simple leg exercises while seated, such as ankle pumps and leg lifts, to stimulate circulation in your lower limbs.

Incorporating walking into your travel plans can be both enjoyable and beneficial. Instead of relying solely on public transportation or taxis, opt to explore your destination on foot whenever possible. Walking tours not only allow you to engage with your surroundings but also provide an excellent way to keep your body moving.

If you're visiting a city, consider using walking apps or guided tours that encourage physical activity while showcasing local attractions.

Another practical tip is to utilize hotel amenities that promote physical activity. Many hotels offer fitness centers, swimming pools, or group exercise classes. Make it a point to dedicate some time each day to these facilities, as even short workouts can significantly impact your overall activity levels.

If your hotel lacks these amenities, look for nearby parks or recreational areas where you can jog or engage in outdoor activities.

Finally, be mindful of your hydration and nutrition while traveling. Staying hydrated is crucial for maintaining overall health, especially during long journeys. Dehydration can exacerbate the risk of blood clots, so drink plenty of water and limit your intake of alcohol and caffeine.

Additionally, opt for healthy snacks like fruits, nuts, and whole grains to keep your energy levels stable, allowing you to remain active and engaged throughout your travels. By implementing these tips, you can enjoy your trips while actively reducing your risk of pulmonary embolism.

Hydration and Nutrition on the Go

Hydration and nutrition are critical factors in maintaining overall health, especially for individuals concerned about pulmonary embolism. When the body is dehydrated, blood becomes thicker, which can increase the risk of clot formation. Proper hydration helps to maintain optimal blood viscosity, supporting healthy circulation.

It is essential to drink adequate fluids throughout the day, particularly when engaged in activities that may lead to fluid loss, such as exercise or travel. Water is often the best choice, but hydrating foods like fruits and vegetables can also contribute significantly to overall fluid intake.

On-the-go lifestyles can make it challenging to prioritize hydration and nutrition. However, planning ahead can make a difference. Carrying a reusable water bottle ensures that you have access to water wherever you are.

It is advisable to aim for a minimum of eight 8-ounce glasses of water daily, adjusting based on activity levels and environmental conditions.

Additionally, incorporating portable snacks that are rich in nutrients, such as nuts, seeds, and whole fruits, can help maintain energy levels and provide essential vitamins and minerals that support cardiovascular health.

In terms of nutrition, a balanced diet plays a vital role in preventing pulmonary embolism. Foods rich in omega-3 fatty acids, such as fatty fish, flaxseeds, and walnuts, can help reduce inflammation and promote healthy blood flow. Leafy greens and other vegetables high in vitamin K are essential for maintaining proper blood clotting mechanisms.

Including a variety of colorful fruits and vegetables in your diet can provide antioxidants that combat oxidative stress, further supporting lung health and overall wellness.

When traveling or facing busy schedules, it is important to be mindful of food choices. Fast food and convenience options often lack the nutrients necessary for optimal health and can contribute to weight gain, which is a risk factor for pulmonary embolism.

Opting for healthier alternatives, such as salads with lean protein, whole grain wraps, or homemade energy bars, can ensure that you are nourishing your body adequately.

Meal prepping can be a useful strategy to ensure you have healthy options readily available, reducing reliance on unhealthy choices when time is limited.

Finally, individuals concerned about pulmonary embolism should be aware of the signs of dehydration and nutritional deficiencies. Symptoms such as fatigue, dizziness, or dry skin can indicate that hydration levels are not sufficient.

Furthermore, being mindful of your diet and recognizing the importance of nutrition in preventing clot formation is crucial. Regular check-ins with healthcare professionals can help tailor dietary choices to individual health needs, ensuring that hydration and nutrition support long-term lung health effectively.

Recognizing Symptoms While Traveling

Traveling can introduce an array of experiences, but it can also pose risks for individuals concerned about pulmonary embolism (PE). Recognizing the symptoms of PE while on the move is essential for prompt action and effective management.

Symptoms may manifest differently in various settings, making it crucial for travelers to remain vigilant. Understanding the signs can significantly influence outcomes, especially when immediate medical attention is required.

One of the most common symptoms of pulmonary embolism is sudden shortness of breath. This may occur unexpectedly, even during routine activities such as walking or climbing stairs. Travelers should be aware that this symptom may not always be accompanied by chest pain, which can lead to misinterpretation of the condition.

If you experience unexpected difficulty in breathing, especially after prolonged periods of immobility, such as long flights or car rides, it is essential to seek medical assistance immediately.

Chest pain is another critical symptom to monitor while traveling. It often presents as a sharp or stabbing sensation that may worsen with deep breaths, coughing, or bending over. Travelers should differentiate this pain from typical muscle strain or discomfort related to travel fatigue.

If chest pain occurs alongside shortness of breath or feels unusual, it is vital to consult a healthcare professional, as these symptoms could indicate a serious condition like PE.

Additionally, travelers should be attentive to any symptoms of rapid heart rate or palpitations. An increased heart rate can occur as the body attempts to compensate for decreased oxygen levels due to a blockage in the pulmonary arteries. This symptom may be accompanied by feelings of anxiety or impending doom.

If you notice a significant change in your heart rate, especially if it is persistent or associated with other symptoms like dizziness or fainting, immediate evaluation by a medical professional is warranted.

Swelling in one leg, particularly if it is accompanied by pain or tenderness, can also signal the presence of a deep vein thrombosis (DVT), which is a precursor to pulmonary embolism. Travelers should keep an eye out for any unilateral swelling or discoloration, especially after extended periods of immobility.

Recognizing these symptoms is vital, as timely intervention can prevent the progression to a pulmonary embolism. Always prioritize your health and seek assistance if you notice any concerning signs while traveling, as early detection is key to managing the risks associated with pulmonary embolism.

How To Prevent Pulmonary Embolism

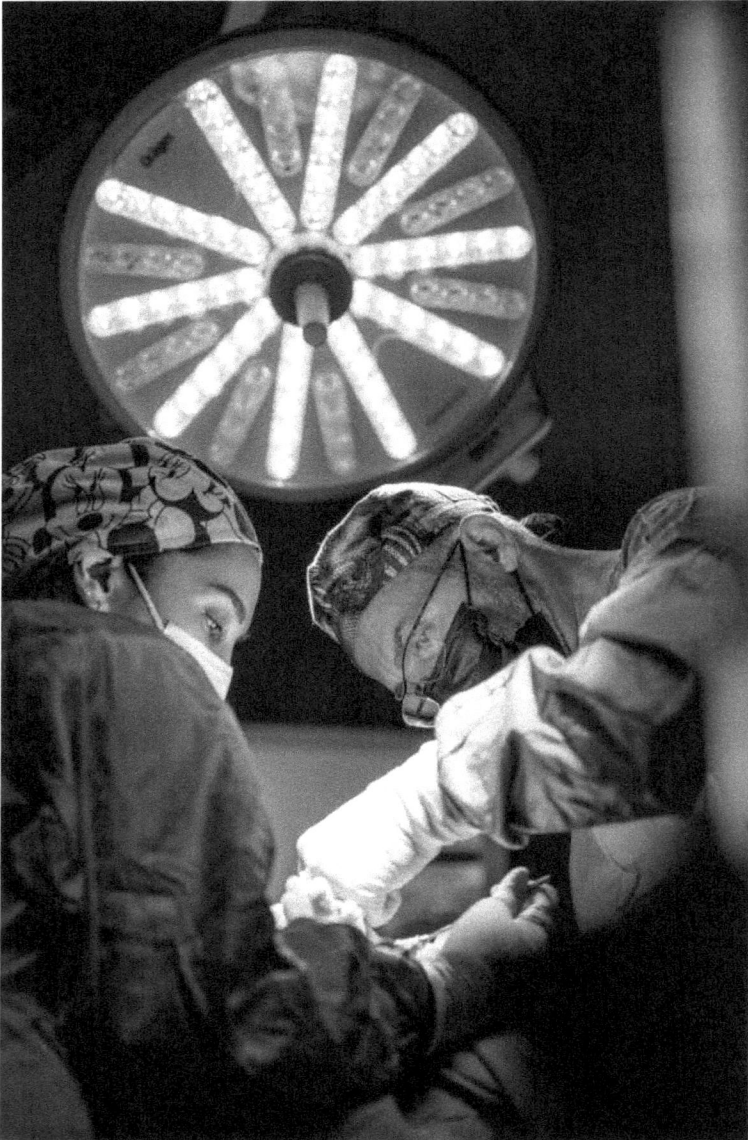

Chapter 6

Special Considerations

Prevention for Post-Surgery Patients

Post-surgery patients are at an increased risk for developing pulmonary embolism (PE) due to factors such as immobility, blood clot formation, and changes in blood flow. Understanding the importance of prevention is crucial for those recovering from surgery.

Implementing specific strategies can significantly reduce the risk of developing a PE, ensuring a smoother recovery process and better overall lung health.

One of the primary strategies for preventing PE in post-surgery patients is to maintain mobility as much as possible. Early ambulation, or getting out of bed and walking shortly after surgery, can help stimulate blood circulation.

It is vital to follow the healthcare provider's recommendations regarding when and how to begin moving. Simple exercises, such as ankle pumps and leg lifts, can also promote blood flow in the legs, minimizing the risk of clot formation.

Compression stockings and devices are another effective preventive measure. Graduated compression stockings apply pressure to the legs, helping to maintain blood flow and reduce swelling. For patients at particularly high risk, pneumatic compression devices may be used to provide intermittent pressure to the legs, enhancing circulation and preventing blood clots. These tools should be used as prescribed by medical professionals to ensure maximum benefit.

Hydration plays a critical role in preventing pulmonary embolism post-surgery. Adequate fluid intake helps to keep the blood from becoming too thick, a condition that can contribute to clot formation. Patients should be encouraged to drink water regularly and avoid excessive consumption of caffeinated or alcoholic beverages, which can lead to dehydration.

Caregivers and family members can support this by providing easy access to fluids and reminding patients to drink throughout the day.

Finally, patients must be vigilant about recognizing the signs and symptoms of pulmonary embolism. Awareness of symptoms such as sudden shortness of breath, chest pain, or coughing up blood is essential for early detection. Patients should feel encouraged to communicate any concerns with their healthcare provider promptly. Regular follow-up appointments and adherence to prescribed anticoagulant therapies, if indicated, are also crucial in mitigating the risk of PE during the recovery period. By combining mobility, compression methods, hydration, and awareness, post-surgery patients can significantly reduce their risk of pulmonary embolism.

Managing Risk During Pregnancy

Managing risk during pregnancy is crucial for the health of both the mother and the baby, particularly when it comes to the prevention of pulmonary embolism (PE). Pregnancy introduces various physiological changes that can increase the risk of thromboembolic events.

Hormonal fluctuations, increased blood volume, and changes in blood flow contribute to a hypercoagulable state. Consequently, understanding and mitigating these risks is essential for pregnant individuals, especially those with a history of clotting disorders, obesity, or other risk factors.

Early prenatal care is vital for identifying individuals at higher risk for pulmonary embolism. Healthcare providers often assess personal and family medical histories to determine risk factors. This evaluation includes screening for conditions such as deep vein thrombosis (DVT) or previous episodes of PE.

Regular consultations with healthcare professionals allow for the development of a personalized care plan that may include lifestyle modifications, medication management, and monitoring protocols to reduce the likelihood of thromboembolic complications during pregnancy.

Lifestyle modifications can significantly lower the risk of developing PE during pregnancy. Maintaining an active lifestyle through regular, moderate exercise can promote healthy circulation and reduce venous stasis. Pregnant individuals should also focus on hydration, as adequate fluid intake helps to prevent blood thickening.

Wearing compression stockings may provide additional support, especially during prolonged periods of sitting or standing, further aiding in venous return and reducing the risk of clot formation.

In some cases, anticoagulant therapy may be warranted for pregnant individuals deemed at high risk for pulmonary embolism. This approach requires careful consideration and monitoring by healthcare providers to balance the benefits of reducing clot risk against potential complications. Low molecular weight heparin is often the preferred choice, as it is considered safe for use during pregnancy.

Close monitoring of both maternal and fetal health is essential to ensure that the treatment plan remains effective and adjusts as needed throughout the pregnancy.

Postpartum care is equally important, as the risk of pulmonary embolism does not dissipate immediately after delivery. The first six weeks following childbirth are particularly critical, as hormonal changes and mobility restrictions can elevate the risk of thromboembolism.

Women should remain vigilant for symptoms such as shortness of breath, chest pain, or leg swelling and seek immediate medical attention if these arise. Ongoing communication with healthcare providers during the postpartum period ensures that any potential issues can be addressed promptly, further safeguarding maternal and fetal well-being.

Guidelines for Individuals with Chronic Illnesses

Individuals with chronic illnesses often face unique challenges that can increase their risk of developing pulmonary embolism (PE). Understanding these challenges is essential for effective prevention and management strategies. One of the primary guidelines is to maintain regular communication with healthcare providers.

This includes discussing any changes in symptoms, medication side effects, or new health concerns. Regular check-ups can help in early detection of potential complications, including those that may contribute to the risk of PE, such as deep vein thrombosis (DVT).

Staying physically active is another critical guideline for those with chronic illnesses. While it may be difficult for some individuals to engage in physical activity due to their health conditions, finding appropriate forms of exercise is vital. Gentle activities such as walking, swimming, or yoga can improve circulation and reduce the risk of blood clots.

It is important to create a personalized exercise plan in consultation with healthcare professionals who understand the individual's specific limitations and health status.

Hydration plays a significant role in preventing blood clots and maintaining overall health. Individuals with chronic illnesses should prioritize staying well-hydrated, as dehydration can increase blood viscosity, making clot formation more likely.

Drinking adequate fluids throughout the day, particularly during warmer weather or after physical activity, is essential. Healthcare providers can offer tailored recommendations on fluid intake based on individual health needs and conditions.

Another guideline focuses on medication management, particularly for those on anticoagulants or other medications that affect blood clotting. It is crucial for individuals to adhere to prescribed medication regimens and to be aware of potential interactions with other medications or supplements.

Regular blood tests may be necessary to monitor the effectiveness of anticoagulants and adjust dosages as needed. Individuals should also be educated about the signs of potential complications, such as unusual bruising or bleeding, which may warrant immediate medical attention.

Lastly, education and awareness about the signs and symptoms of pulmonary embolism are vital. Individuals with chronic illnesses should be knowledgeable about the warning signs, such as sudden shortness of breath, chest pain, and coughing up blood.

Prompt recognition and response to these symptoms can significantly impact outcomes. Participating in support groups or educational sessions can enhance understanding and empower individuals to take proactive steps in their health management, ultimately reducing the risk of pulmonary embolism.

How To Prevent Pulmonary Embolism

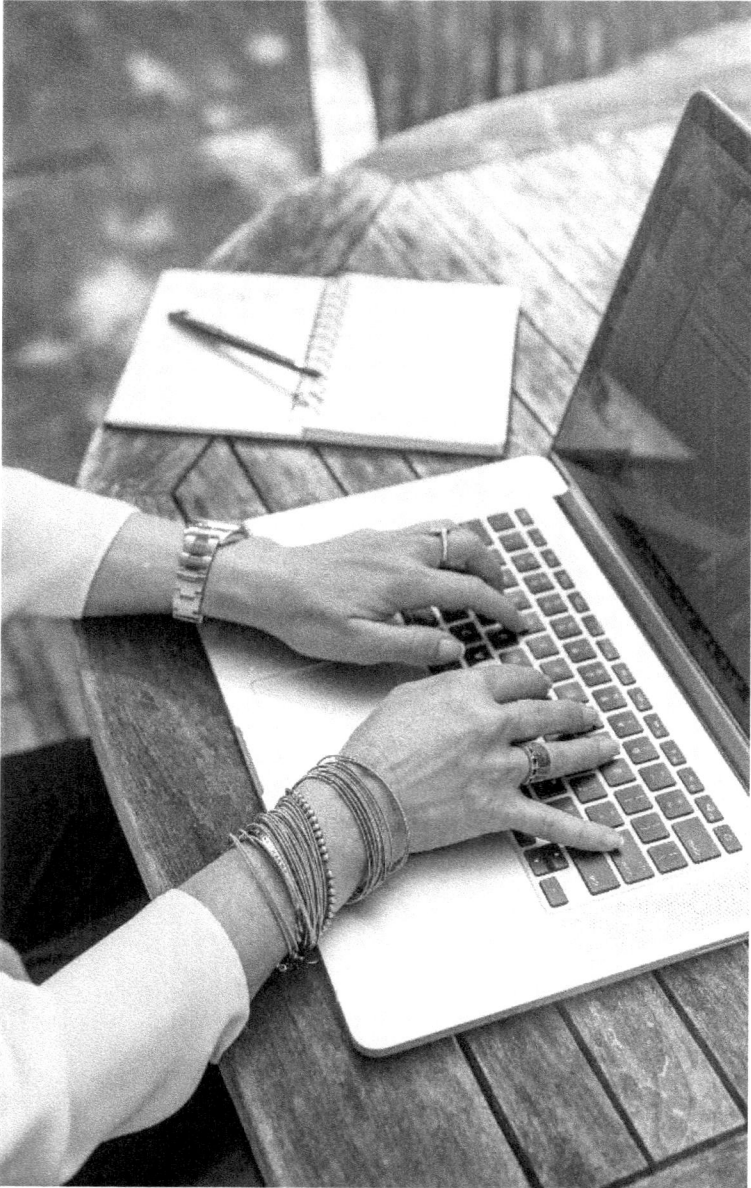

Chapter 7

Educating Yourself and Others

Recognizing the Signs and Symptoms

Recognizing the signs and symptoms of pulmonary embolism (PE) is crucial for timely intervention and prevention. Understanding these indicators can empower individuals to seek medical attention promptly, potentially saving lives. The most common symptoms of PE include sudden shortness of breath, chest pain, and coughing, which may sometimes produce blood. These symptoms can arise suddenly and may vary in intensity, making it essential to remain vigilant if they appear.

Sudden shortness of breath is often the most striking symptom of a pulmonary embolism. This can occur at rest or during physical activity and may feel like a choking sensation or an inability to catch one's breath.

Individuals may also experience increased heart rate and a sense of anxiety, which can exacerbate the feeling of breathlessness. It is essential to recognize that this symptom may not always be associated with a pre-existing respiratory condition, making it a critical sign to monitor.

Chest pain associated with pulmonary embolism can manifest as a sharp or stabbing sensation, often worsening with deep breaths, coughing, or bending over. Some individuals may mistake this pain for a heart attack or other cardiac issue, complicating the recognition of PE.

The pain may be localized or radiate to the shoulder, neck, or jaw. Regardless of its presentation, any unexplained chest pain, particularly when accompanied by other symptoms, should prompt immediate medical evaluation.

Coughing is another symptom that may indicate a pulmonary embolism, particularly if it produces bloody sputum. This hemoptysis occurs when a blood clot affects blood vessels in the lungs, leading to bleeding. While coughing can be attributed to various conditions, the presence of blood should never be overlooked.

It is critical to differentiate between a mild cough and one that raises blood, as the latter may indicate a serious underlying issue requiring urgent care.

Additional signs such as swelling in one leg, warmth, and tenderness may also indicate a deep vein thrombosis (DVT), which can lead to pulmonary embolism if a clot dislodges and travels to the lungs. This swelling is typically unilateral and can occur without any visible injury. Recognizing these symptoms early can lead to prompt treatment and significantly reduce the risk of developing a PE. Awareness and education about these signs can play a vital role in prevention efforts and improving lung health for those at risk.

Communicating with Healthcare Providers

Effective communication with healthcare providers is essential for anyone concerned about pulmonary embolism (PE). Establishing a clear line of dialogue can significantly enhance your understanding of the condition, its risks, and preventive measures.

When you engage with healthcare professionals, it is crucial to express your concerns openly, ask questions, and share your medical history. By doing so, you enable your provider to offer tailored advice and strategies that are specific to your health needs.

Before your appointment, prepare a list of questions or topics you want to discuss. This preparation can help ensure that you cover all your concerns during the visit. Questions may include inquiries about your risk factors for PE, the signs and symptoms to watch for, and the specific lifestyle changes you can implement to reduce your risk.

Additionally, understanding the role of medications, such as anticoagulants, in both prevention and treatment can be an important aspect of your discussion.

During the consultation, it's important to be honest about your lifestyle, including your activity level, diet, and any existing medical conditions. Providers rely on accurate information to assess your risk for pulmonary embolism effectively.

If you have a history of blood clots or other related conditions, make sure to inform your healthcare provider. This information can lead to more proactive monitoring and personalized prevention strategies that align with your unique situation.

After your appointment, take the time to review the information provided. If there were terms or concepts that were unclear, consider following up with your provider for clarification.

Many healthcare facilities offer patient portals that allow you to access your health information and communicate with your provider. Utilize these resources to ask additional questions or express any ongoing concerns. Understanding your treatment plan and the rationale behind it is vital in adhering to preventive measures.

Lastly, consider bringing a family member or friend to your appointments. Having an additional person can help you remember important details and provide emotional support. They can also assist in asking questions or voicing concerns that you might overlook.

Remember, effective communication is a two-way street; being proactive and engaged in your healthcare discussions can empower you to take control of your lung health and significantly reduce your risk of pulmonary embolism.

Raising Awareness in Your Community

Raising awareness in your community about pulmonary embolism (PE) is crucial for prevention and early intervention. Many people are unaware of the risk factors, symptoms, and the importance of seeking immediate medical attention. By educating those around you, you can help reduce the incidence of this potentially life-threatening condition. Community awareness can lead to early diagnosis and treatment, which significantly improves outcomes for those affected by PE.

One effective way to raise awareness is through educational workshops and seminars. Partnering with local health organizations, hospitals, or community centers can provide a platform for disseminating information.

These events can cover topics such as the risk factors associated with PE, including prolonged immobility, certain medical conditions, and lifestyle choices. By providing clear and accessible information, you can empower individuals to recognize their own risk and take preventive measures.

Social media campaigns are another powerful tool for spreading awareness. Utilizing platforms like Facebook, Twitter, and Instagram can help reach a broader audience. Sharing informative posts, infographics, and personal stories can engage the community and encourage discussions about pulmonary embolism. Creating a dedicated page or group focused on PE can foster a supportive environment where individuals can ask questions, share experiences, and learn from one another.

Involving local healthcare professionals can enhance awareness initiatives. Hosting Q&A sessions with doctors, nurses, or specialists can provide valuable insights into pulmonary embolism. These professionals can clarify misconceptions, discuss the importance of regular check-ups, and emphasize the role of lifestyle changes in prevention.

By having trusted figures in the community participate in these events, you can increase credibility and encourage more people to attend and seek out information.

Finally, consider organizing community health fairs or screening events that focus on lung health and PE prevention. Offering free or low-cost screenings for risk factors such as high blood pressure and blood clotting disorders can identify individuals who may need further evaluation. These events can also include educational booths, demonstrations, and materials that promote awareness and prevention strategies. Engaging the community in this way creates a proactive approach to health and encourages individuals to prioritize their well-being.

Resources for Ongoing Education

To effectively prevent pulmonary embolism, ongoing education is crucial for individuals at risk. Understanding the condition, its causes, and preventive measures can significantly empower individuals to take charge of their lung health.

A variety of resources are available to help those concerned about pulmonary embolism stay informed. By utilizing these resources, individuals can enhance their knowledge and make informed decisions about their health.

One primary resource is reliable online platforms dedicated to pulmonary health and disease prevention. Websites from reputable organizations such as the American Lung Association and the Centers for Disease Control and Prevention offer comprehensive information about pulmonary embolism. These sites provide insights into risk factors, symptoms, and preventive strategies, ensuring that individuals have access to current and evidence-based information.

Additionally, many of these platforms offer newsletters and updates that can keep individuals informed about the latest research and developments in lung health.

Books and publications also serve as valuable resources for ongoing education. Numerous titles focus on pulmonary health, prevention strategies, and lifestyle modifications that can reduce the risk of pulmonary embolism. These books often feature personal anecdotes, expert advice, and practical tips that readers can implement in their daily lives.

By exploring various publications, individuals can find guidance tailored to their specific concerns and circumstances, making it easier to adopt healthier practices.

Participating in support groups and community programs can enhance education and awareness regarding pulmonary embolism. Many hospitals and health organizations host workshops, seminars, and support groups where individuals can learn from healthcare professionals and share experiences with others facing similar challenges.

These interactions not only provide essential information but also foster a sense of community, encouraging individuals to remain proactive about their health and seek help when needed.

Finally, consulting healthcare professionals is an indispensable resource for ongoing education. Regular check-ups and discussions with doctors or specialists can provide personalized insights into individual risk factors and preventive measures. Healthcare providers can recommend appropriate lifestyle changes, screenings, and treatments tailored to a person's specific health profile, ensuring a comprehensive approach to preventing pulmonary embolism.

By establishing a strong partnership with healthcare professionals, individuals can stay informed and proactive in maintaining their lung health.

How To Prevent Pulmonary Embolism

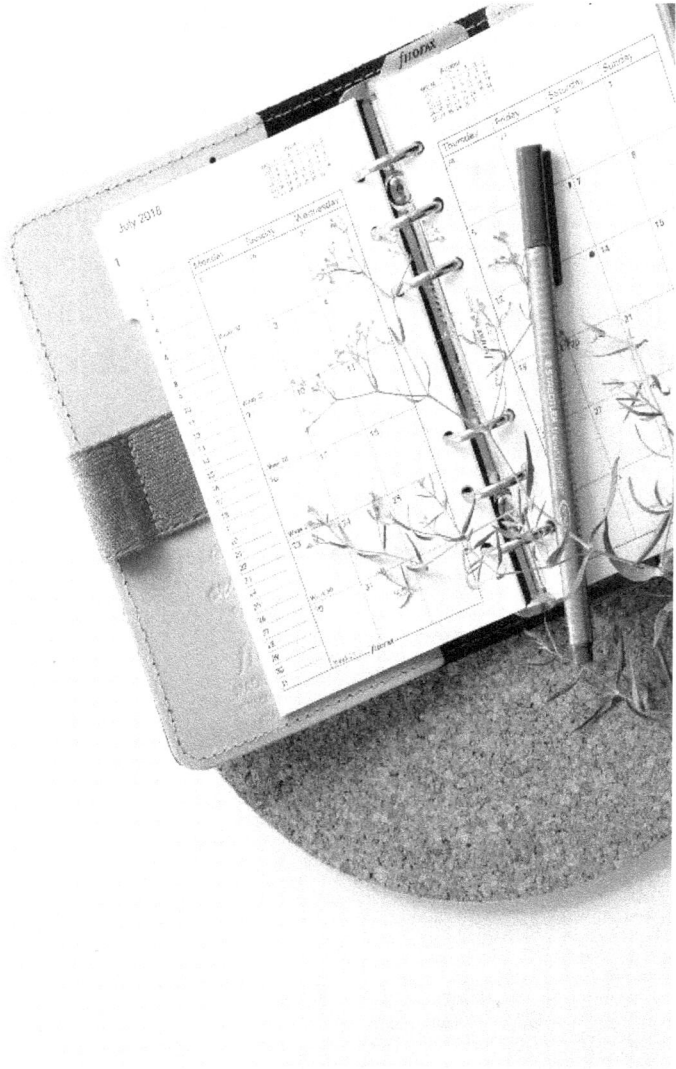

Chapter 8

Developing a Personal Prevention Plan

Assessing Your Individual Risk

Assessing your individual risk for pulmonary embolism (PE) is a critical step in prevention. Understanding the factors that contribute to your likelihood of developing this potentially life-threatening condition can empower you to make informed decisions about your health.

Risk assessment involves evaluating various elements, including personal medical history, lifestyle choices, and genetic predispositions. By gaining insight into your unique risk profile, you can take proactive measures to mitigate the threat of PE.

Several medical conditions are known to increase the risk of pulmonary embolism. Individuals with a history of deep vein thrombosis (DVT), certain cancers, or heart disease are at heightened risk.

Additionally, those who undergo surgical procedures, particularly orthopedic surgeries, should be aware of their vulnerability. It is crucial to discuss your medical history with your healthcare provider, as they can offer personalized advice on how to lower your risk based on your specific health circumstances.

Lifestyle factors also play a significant role in the risk of developing PE. Sedentary behavior, such as prolonged sitting during long travel or extended periods of immobility, can lead to blood clots. Similarly, smoking is a well-established risk factor that can contribute to vascular issues and increase the likelihood of clot formation.

Regular physical activity, a balanced diet, and avoiding tobacco can substantially reduce your risk. Being mindful of these lifestyle choices is essential for maintaining overall cardiovascular health.

Genetic predisposition is another important aspect of risk assessment. Certain inherited conditions, such as Factor V Leiden or prothrombin gene mutation, can increase the likelihood of clot formation.

If you have a family history of clotting disorders, it is advisable to discuss this with your doctor, as they may recommend further evaluation or preventative measures. Genetic testing can provide clarity and assist in creating a tailored prevention strategy.

Finally, assessing your individual risk for pulmonary embolism involves a comprehensive approach that includes awareness of both medical and lifestyle factors. Regular check-ups with healthcare professionals are vital for monitoring any changes in your condition. By actively engaging in your health management, you can identify potential risks early on and implement strategies to prevent pulmonary embolism. Remember that understanding your risk is a powerful tool in safeguarding your lung health and overall well-being.

Setting Goals for Better Lung Health

Setting goals for better lung health is a crucial step in preventing pulmonary embolism, a serious condition that can lead to life-threatening complications.

Establishing clear and achievable goals allows individuals to focus on specific actions that promote optimal lung function and overall well-being. By identifying personal health objectives, individuals can create a roadmap that not only supports lung health but also reduces the risk of developing conditions that may lead to pulmonary embolism.

One effective approach to goal setting is the SMART criteria: goals should be Specific, Measurable, Achievable, Relevant, and Time-bound. For instance, instead of setting a vague goal like "improve lung health," a SMART goal could be "walk for 30 minutes five times a week for the next three months."

This specific target encourages regular physical activity, which is vital for maintaining healthy circulation and preventing blood clots, a key factor in the risk of pulmonary embolism.

In addition to physical activity, individuals should also focus on nutrition as part of their lung health goals. A balanced diet rich in fruits, vegetables, whole grains, and lean proteins can provide essential nutrients that support respiratory function.

Setting a goal to incorporate at least one serving of leafy greens into each meal or to drink a certain amount of water daily can help ensure proper hydration and nutrient intake. These dietary changes can improve overall health and may also enhance blood flow, further reducing the risk of clot formation.

Monitoring progress is essential in the goal-setting process. Keeping a journal or using a mobile app to track activities, dietary choices, and overall well-being can provide valuable insights. Regularly reviewing these records allows individuals to assess their progress toward lung health goals and make necessary adjustments.

This reflective practice not only fosters accountability but also helps individuals stay motivated and engaged in their health journey, reinforcing the importance of each small step taken.

Lastly, it is vital to seek support from healthcare professionals and loved ones when setting and pursuing health goals. Engaging in discussions with doctors, nutritionists, or respiratory therapists can provide tailored advice and resources that enhance the goal-setting process.

Additionally, sharing goals with family and friends can create a support system that encourages accountability and offers motivation. By fostering a collaborative approach to lung health, individuals can significantly reduce their risk of pulmonary embolism while promoting a healthier lifestyle overall.

Tracking Your Progress

Tracking your progress in preventing pulmonary embolism is a crucial step in managing your lung health. This involves monitoring various aspects of your health and lifestyle to identify areas of improvement and ensure that you are adhering to preventive measures.

Keeping a record of your activities, symptoms, and responses to treatments can help you and your healthcare provider make informed decisions about your care. By establishing a systematic approach to tracking your progress, you can gain insights into your health and take proactive steps to minimize your risk.

One effective method for tracking your progress is to maintain a health journal. In this journal, you can document daily activities, exercise routines, and any symptoms you experience. Noting changes in weight, diet, and medication adherence will also provide valuable information.

This practice not only helps in identifying patterns but also serves as a motivational tool. You may find that recording small victories, such as completing a week of regular physical activity or making healthier food choices, reinforces positive behavior and encourages continued commitment to your health goals.

Utilizing technology can enhance your ability to track progress. There are various apps and wearable devices designed to monitor physical activity, heart rate, and even blood oxygen levels. These tools can provide real-time data that helps you understand how your body is responding to your efforts.

For instance, consistent tracking of your physical activity can reveal trends, such as improvements in endurance or increased mobility. Moreover, some apps allow you to set reminders for medication and hydration, ensuring that you stay on top of your preventive measures.

Regular medical check-ups are another essential component of tracking your progress. These appointments provide an opportunity for healthcare professionals to assess your lung health, evaluate any risk factors, and adjust your treatment plan as necessary. During these visits, you can discuss your health journal findings and any data collected from technology tools, allowing for a collaborative approach to your care.

Your healthcare provider can also perform tests, such as blood work or imaging, to monitor your condition and detect any early signs of complications.

Finally, reflecting on your progress regularly is vital. Set aside time each month to review your health journal and any data collected through apps or devices. Consider what strategies have been effective and which areas may need improvement.

This reflection not only helps in adjusting your approach but also reinforces a sense of accountability. By actively engaging in the process of tracking your progress, you empower yourself to take control of your lung health and reduce the risk of pulmonary embolism, ultimately leading to a healthier and more fulfilling life.

Seeking Support and Accountability

Seeking support and accountability is a crucial aspect of preventing pulmonary embolism, especially for individuals who are at higher risk. Engaging with a community can provide not only emotional support but also practical resources and knowledge.

This can include support groups, online forums, or even local health organizations that focus on lung health. Sharing experiences and strategies with others who have similar concerns can empower individuals, making them feel less isolated in their journey toward better lung health.

Establishing a strong support network can also facilitate accountability. When people share their goals with others, they are more likely to stay committed to those goals. This could mean regularly discussing lifestyle changes, medication adherence, or exercise routines with friends, family, or support group members.

Accountability partners can motivate each other to maintain healthy behaviors and remind one another of the importance of these actions in preventing pulmonary embolism. This shared commitment can lead to healthier habits and a greater sense of community.

In addition to peer support, seeking professional guidance is essential. Healthcare providers can offer tailored advice on risk factors associated with pulmonary embolism and strategies for prevention. Regular check-ins with a physician or a specialist can help individuals stay informed about their health status and adjust their prevention strategies as necessary.

Medical professionals can also provide educational materials and resources that can deepen understanding of the condition, which is vital for effective prevention.

Utilizing technology can further enhance support and accountability efforts. Mobile applications and online platforms designed for health tracking can help individuals monitor their activities, medications, and any symptoms they may experience.

These tools can serve as reminders for necessary lifestyle changes, such as increasing physical activity or maintaining hydration, both of which play a significant role in lung health. By integrating technology into their prevention plan, individuals can stay engaged and proactive in their approach to avoiding pulmonary embolism.

Finally, fostering a culture of open communication within families and communities about lung health can contribute to prevention efforts. Discussing the risks and signs of pulmonary embolism can raise awareness and encourage others to take preventive measures seriously.

By creating an environment where individuals feel comfortable sharing their health concerns and experiences, communities can collectively work toward minimizing the risks associated with pulmonary embolism. This collaborative spirit not only enhances individual accountability but also promotes a broader understanding of the importance of lung health in preventing serious conditions.

How To Prevent Pulmonary Embolism

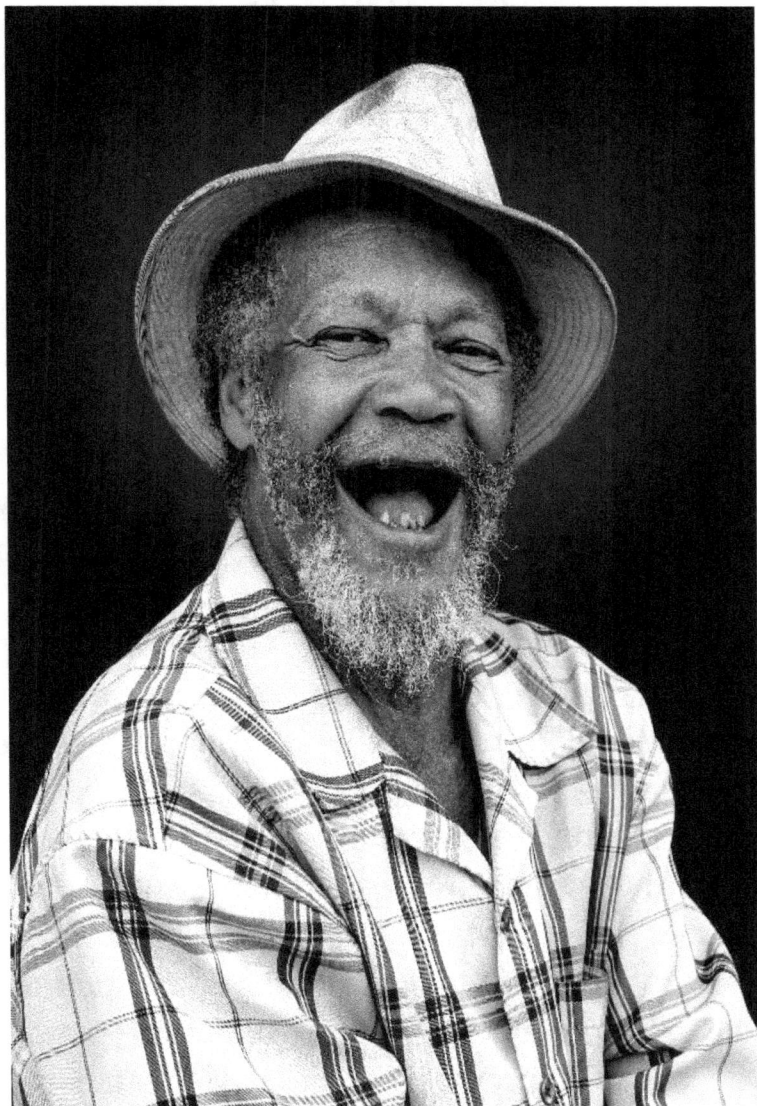

Chapter 9

Conclusion and Next Steps

Recap of Key Concepts

Understanding pulmonary embolism (PE) is crucial for those concerned about their lung health. PE occurs when a blood clot travels to the lungs, blocking a pulmonary artery and potentially leading to severe complications. Recognizing the risk factors associated with PE is the first step in prevention.

These risk factors include prolonged immobility, certain medical conditions such as heart disease or cancer, and the use of hormonal therapy. By identifying these risks, individuals can take proactive measures to minimize their chances of experiencing a PE.

Awareness of the symptoms of pulmonary embolism is equally important. Common symptoms include sudden shortness of breath, chest pain that may worsen with deep breaths, rapid heart rate, and coughing up blood.

Knowing these signs enables individuals to seek immediate medical attention, which is critical for reducing the risk of serious outcomes. Early detection can lead to timely treatment, which may involve anticoagulants or other interventions to dissolve the clot and restore blood flow to the lungs.

Preventive strategies play a vital role in safeguarding lung health. Lifestyle modifications such as regular physical activity, maintaining a healthy weight, and staying hydrated can significantly decrease the risk of blood clots. For those who are at higher risk, such as individuals recovering from surgery or those with limited mobility, preventive measures might include the use of compression stockings or anticoagulant medications. Engaging in these practices consistently can create a protective barrier against the development of PE.

Education about the importance of regular medical check-ups and screenings cannot be overstated. Health professionals can provide personalized advice and monitor any underlying conditions that may predispose an individual to pulmonary embolism.

Regular assessments can help identify issues early, allowing for timely interventions. This proactive approach not only aids in prevention but also promotes overall lung health, ensuring that individuals can enjoy a better quality of life.

Finally, fostering a supportive community can enhance awareness and prevention efforts. Engaging with others who share similar concerns can lead to the exchange of valuable information and resources. Support groups and educational workshops can empower individuals with knowledge about pulmonary embolism and its prevention. By creating an environment where open discussions about lung health are encouraged, individuals can better equip themselves to take charge of their health and reduce their risk of pulmonary embolism.

The Future of Lung Health Research

The future of lung health research is poised to bring transformative advancements that could significantly improve prevention strategies for pulmonary embolism (PE) and enhance overall lung health.

Innovations in technology, including artificial intelligence and machine learning, are expected to play a pivotal role in early detection and risk assessment. By analyzing large datasets, researchers can identify patterns and risk factors associated with PE, leading to more personalized prevention strategies tailored to individual patients. This could ultimately reduce the incidence of PE and improve patient outcomes.

In addition to technological advancements, the development of new biomarkers holds promise for lung health research. Biomarkers are biological indicators that can signal the presence of disease or the risk of developing one.

Researchers are actively investigating various biomarkers that could predict clot formation or identify individuals at higher risk for PE. Early identification of those at risk may allow for timely interventions, such as anticoagulant therapy or lifestyle modifications, to prevent the occurrence of pulmonary embolism.

Furthermore, the field of genomics is making strides in understanding the genetic predispositions associated with lung diseases, including PE. By studying the genetic profiles of individuals with a history of pulmonary embolism, researchers aim to uncover hereditary factors that contribute to the condition.

This genetic insight can lead to targeted prevention efforts, as well as the development of new therapeutic approaches that consider a patient's genetic background. Improved understanding of these genetic links is essential for advancing personalized medicine in the context of lung health.

Collaboration among researchers, healthcare providers, and patients is also crucial for advancing lung health research. Engaging patients in research initiatives can provide valuable insights into their experiences and challenges, ensuring that studies address real-world issues. Additionally, multi-disciplinary collaborations can lead to holistic approaches that integrate various aspects of lung health, including behavioral, environmental, and medical factors.

Such partnerships can facilitate the development of comprehensive prevention programs that are more effective in reducing the risk of pulmonary embolism.

Finally, public awareness and education about lung health and pulmonary embolism are vital components of future research initiatives. As knowledge about risk factors, symptoms, and prevention strategies expands, it is essential to disseminate this information to the public.

Initiatives that focus on educating communities about the importance of lung health, the signs of PE, and the steps to take for prevention can empower individuals to take control of their health.

Increased awareness can lead to earlier diagnosis and intervention, ultimately reducing the burden of pulmonary embolism and improving lung health for future generations.

Encouragement for Ongoing Commitment to Prevention

Ongoing commitment to prevention is essential for reducing the risk of pulmonary embolism (PE), a serious condition that can have life-threatening consequences. Understanding the factors that contribute to PE can empower individuals to take proactive steps toward maintaining their lung health.

Engaging in regular discussions with healthcare providers about personal risk factors, such as obesity, prolonged immobility, or a history of blood clots, can help tailor prevention strategies that are specific to individual needs. This dialogue is crucial for staying informed about the latest research and recommendations in PE prevention.

Implementing lifestyle changes plays a significant role in reducing the risk of pulmonary embolism. Regular physical activity is one of the most effective preventive measures. Engaging in moderate exercise, such as walking, swimming, or cycling, helps improve blood circulation and reduces the likelihood of blood clots forming in the legs.

Additionally, maintaining a healthy weight through balanced nutrition can lower the risk factors associated with PE. Individuals should consider incorporating more fruits, vegetables, whole grains, and lean proteins into their diets while minimizing processed foods and sugars.

For those with pre-existing medical conditions or risk factors for clot development, adhering to prescribed medications is vital. Anticoagulants, commonly known as blood thinners, can significantly decrease the likelihood of clot formation in at-risk populations.

It is essential for individuals to understand their medications, including how they work and potential side effects. Regular follow-ups with healthcare providers to monitor health status and medication effectiveness are important in ensuring ongoing protection against pulmonary embolism.

Education and awareness are fundamental components of prevention. Individuals should familiarize themselves with the symptoms of pulmonary embolism, such as sudden shortness of breath, chest pain, or coughing up blood.

Recognizing these signs early can lead to prompt medical attention, which is critical for improving outcomes. Community resources, such as educational workshops or support groups, can offer valuable information and foster a sense of shared responsibility among those concerned about pulmonary embolism.

Lastly, fostering a long-term commitment to prevention requires a supportive environment. Family and friends can play a key role in encouraging healthy behaviors and reminding individuals to prioritize their lung health. Creating a routine that incorporates preventive measures, such as regular exercise and nutritious meals, can reinforce positive habits.

By cultivating a culture of health and awareness, individuals can take significant strides in minimizing their risk of pulmonary embolism and promoting overall well-being.

Final Thoughts on Living a Healthier Life

Living a healthier life requires a multifaceted approach that emphasizes prevention, awareness, and proactive measures. For individuals concerned about pulmonary embolism, it is crucial to understand that lifestyle choices significantly influence overall lung health.

Engaging in regular physical activity, maintaining a balanced diet, and staying hydrated can enhance circulation and reduce the risk of blood clots. Simple changes, such as incorporating more fruits and vegetables into meals and participating in moderate exercise, can have profound effects on lung function and overall well-being.

Awareness of personal health conditions is another essential aspect of preventing pulmonary embolism. Individuals with risk factors, such as obesity, prolonged inactivity, or a history of clotting disorders, should monitor their health closely. Regular check-ups with healthcare providers can help identify potential issues before they escalate.

Additionally, understanding the signs and symptoms of pulmonary embolism, such as sudden shortness of breath, chest pain, or rapid heart rate, can lead to timely medical intervention and potentially save lives.

Education plays a pivotal role in prevention. Knowledge about the mechanisms of pulmonary embolism, including how blood clots form and travel to the lungs, empowers individuals to make informed decisions regarding their health. This includes understanding the importance of anticoagulant medications for those at high risk and the need for strategies such as compression stockings during long flights or extended periods of immobility.

By staying informed, individuals can actively participate in their health management and reduce their risk of developing complications.

Social support and community resources also contribute to a healthier lifestyle. Engaging with support groups or health-focused communities can provide motivation and accountability.

Sharing experiences and strategies with others who face similar health concerns fosters a sense of belonging and encourages positive lifestyle changes.

Furthermore, accessing community programs that promote physical activity, nutrition education, and smoking cessation can enhance individual efforts to maintain lung health.

In conclusion, living a healthier life, particularly concerning the prevention of pulmonary embolism, encompasses a commitment to making informed choices, staying active, and seeking support. By prioritizing health, being vigilant about risk factors, and utilizing available resources, individuals can significantly reduce their likelihood of experiencing pulmonary embolism.

This proactive approach not only safeguards lung health but also enriches overall quality of life, enabling individuals to thrive and enjoy their daily activities with greater vitality.

Author Notes & Acknowledgments

First and foremost, I would like to express my deepest gratitude to the people who inspired and supported me throughout the journey of writing this book. This project would not have been possible without their unwavering belief in me and their invaluable contributions.

To my wife, thank you for your constant encouragement and understanding. Your love and support have been my anchor during the challenging times of researching and writing this book. Your belief in my ability to make a difference in people's lives has been my driving force.

I would also like to disclose that this book contains some renewed artificial intelligence-generated content. I really appreciate very recent technological innovation by outstanding scientists and of course our reader's understanding.

Lastly, I want to express my deepest gratitude to the readers of this book. I sincerely hope the strategies and methods outlined within these pages will provide you with the knowledge and tools needed to truly make your life much better. Your commitment to seeking any good solutions and willingness to explore multiple methods is commendable.

Author Bio

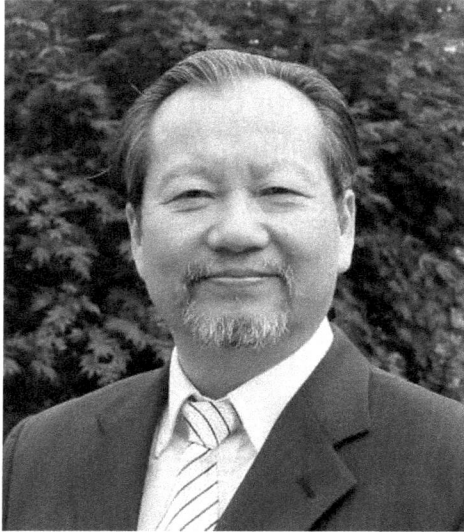

Johnson Wu earned his MD in 1982. With over 40 years of clinical experience, he has worked in hospitals in Zhejiang and Shanghai, China, as well as the Royal Marsden Hospital (part of Imperial College) in London, UK. Upon the recommendation of Sir Aaron Klug, the president of The Royal Society and a Nobel Prize winner in Chemistry, Dr. Wu was honorably awarded a British Royal Society Fellowship. He has published over 100 medical books in many countries and currently practices medicine in Canada.

www.ingramcontent.com/pod-product-compliance
Lightning Source LLC
Chambersburg PA
CBHW060244030426
42335CB00014B/1590